THE **NECK** BOOK

London: TSO

First published 2004
Ninth impression 2011

Single copies ISBN 978 0 11 703321 4 Price £1.50

Discounts apply for larger quantities. Call 0870 600 5522

Pack of 10 copies ISBN 978 0 11 703354 2

1-5 packs	Price £13 per pack
6-19 packs	Price £11 per pack
Over 20 packs	Price on application

Also available from TSO

- Back Book (ISBN 978 0 11 702949 1) offering advice to those with lower back pain
- 'Get Back Active' (ISBN 978 0 11 7039360) a DVD based on the Back Book giving practical guidance on handling back pain
- 'The Whiplash Book' (ISBN 978 0 11 702029 0) offering advice on how to deal with a whiplash injury - based on the latest research

The help and advice from colleagues too numerous to mention is gratefully acknowledged

Printed in the United Kingdom by The Stationery Office
J002465587 C60 07/11 13380

A BETTER APPROACH TO NECK PAIN

Neck pain is very common and can cause a great deal of misery but, fortunately, serious or permanent damage is rare. There has been a change in thinking about neck pain and we now deal with it in a different way. This booklet sets out the facts and shows you how to get better as quickly as possible. It is based on the latest research.

What you do about neck pain yourself is usually more important than the exact diagnosis or treatment.

Acute neck pain can be distressing. Even a minor neck strain can be very painful and it's natural to think that something terrible might have happened. But stop and look at the facts:

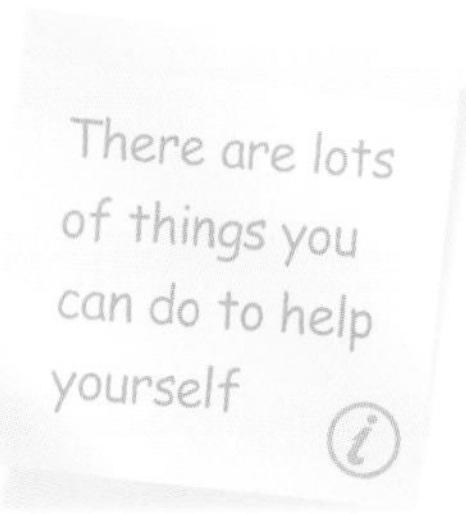

NECK FACTS

- Neck pain is rarely due to any serious disease.
- The acute pain usually improves within days or a few weeks, at least enough to get on with your life.
- Sometimes aches and pains can last for quite a long time, or come and go. But that still doesn't mean it's serious. Most people can get going quite quickly, even while they still have some pain. Between attacks most people return to normal activities with little if any pain.

Serious or permanent damage is rare

- What you do in the early stages is very important. Rest for more than a day or two usually does not help and may actually prolong pain and disability.
- Your neck is designed for movement: it needs movement - a lot of movement. The sooner you get moving and doing your ordinary activities as normally as possible, the sooner you will feel better.
- The people who cope best with neck pain are those who stay active and get on with life despite the pain.

The sooner you get on with your life - the sooner you will feel better

CAUSES OF NECK PAIN

Your neck is strong. Like the rest of your spine, your neck is made of solid bony blocks joined by discs to give it strength and flexibility. It is reinforced by strong ligaments, and surrounded by large and powerful muscles that protect it. Most simple neck strains do not cause any lasting damage.

Despite what you might have heard:

- Very few people with neck pain have a disc problem or a trapped nerve. Minor nerve irritation usually gets better by itself. Neck pain hardly ever needs surgery.
- X-rays and MRI scans can detect serious spinal conditions, but they don't usually help in ordinary neck pain. They may even be misleading. Very often the scans of people without neck pain show what doctors sometimes call 'degenerative changes', which may sound alarming but really just refers to normal changes with age - just like grey hair. 'Degenerative change' does not mean you have damage or arthritis.

Your doctor or therapist will often not be able to pinpoint the source of the pain. It may be frustrating not to know exactly what is wrong. Actually, in another way it's good news - you do not have anything serious.

Most neck pain comes from the working parts of your neck - the muscles, ligaments, and small joints. Your neck is simply not moving and working as it should. You can think of it being seized up. So what you should do is get it moving. This stimulates its natural ability to recover. And don't worry if your neck creaks a bit when you move it. Again, that's normal. All joints make sounds – they just seem louder when they're near your ears!

Some people with neck pain may also get headache, arm or chest pain, or mild pins and needles. That's common, and does not mean a trapped nerve. Those symptoms generally settle along with the neck pain.

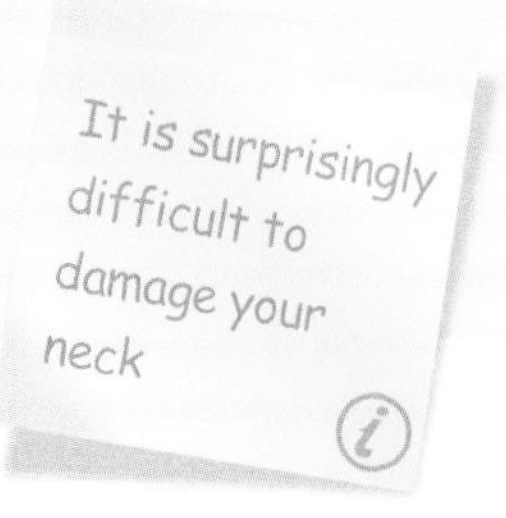

REST OR STAY ACTIVE?

The old fashioned treatment was rest and immobilisation. Some people with back or neck pain went to bed or used a collar for months on end, just waiting for the pain to disappear. We now know that rest for more than a day or two is the worst possible treatment, because in the long term it actually prolongs the pain:

- You get stiff.
- Your muscles get weak.
- You lose physical fitness.
- You get depressed.
- The pain feels worse.
- It is harder and harder to get going again.

No wonder it didn't work! The message is now clear: PROLONGED INACTIVITY IS BAD FOR NECK PAIN.

You may be limited in how much you can do when the pain is bad. You might even be forced to rest at the start. But only for a day or two. Rest is not a treatment – it's simply a short-term consequence of the pain. The most important thing is to get moving again as soon as you can.

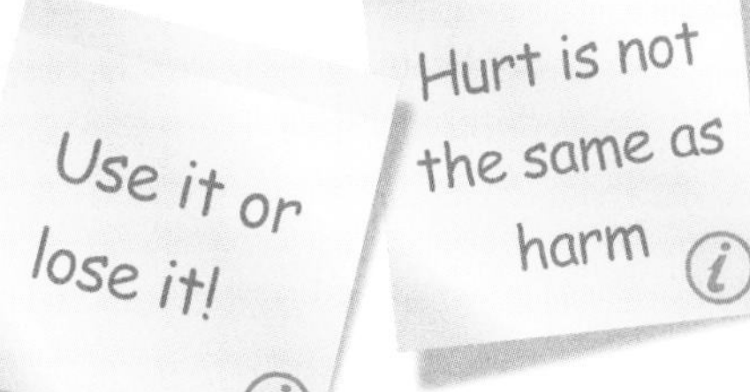

ACTIVITY IS GOOD

MOVEMENT IS GOOD FOR YOU – AND FOR YOUR NECK

Your whole body must keep active to stay healthy. It thrives on use.

Regular physical activity:

- Gives you stronger bones.
- Develops your muscles.
- Keeps you supple.
- Makes you fit.
- Makes you feel good.
- Releases natural chemicals that reduce the pain.

Even when your neck is painful, you can make a start without putting too much stress on it.

- Simple neck exercises.
- Keep fit exercises.
- Yoga (but avoid headstands!).
- Walking.
- In fact, most daily activities and hobbies.

Exercise gets your neck moving again by stretching tight muscles and joints, and stops the working parts stiffening up.

Different things suit different people. Experiment - find what works best for you and your neck. Your goal is to get moving and steadily increase your level of activity. Do a bit more each day. It helps to do things you enjoy.

Getting stiff joints and muscles working can be painful. Athletes accept that when they start training, their muscles can hurt and they have to work through the pain. But that does not mean they are doing any damage. So don't worry if exercise makes you a bit sore at first – that's usually a sign you are actually making progress! As you get fully active, the pain should ease off.

Nobody pretends it's easy. Painkillers and other treatments can help to control the pain to let you get started, but you still have to do the work. There is no other way. You have a straight choice: rest and get worse, or get active and recover.

Do not fall into the trap of thinking it will be easier in a week or two, next month, next year. It won't! The longer you put it off, the harder it will be to get going again. The faster you get back to normal activities and back to work the better - even if you still have some restrictions.

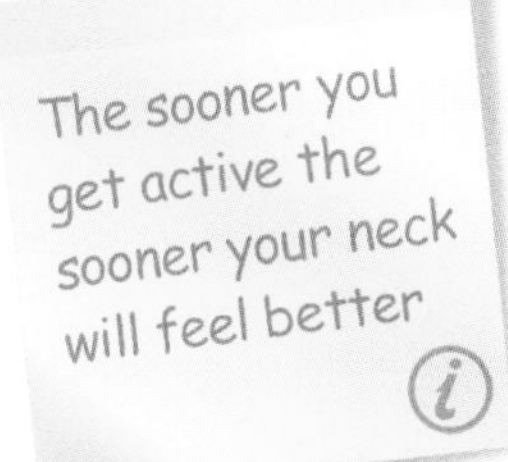

DEALING WITH ACUTE NECK PAIN

Most people usually manage to deal with neck pain themselves:

- Use something to control the pain.
- Modify your activities for a time, if necessary.
- Do neck exercises – some good ones are shown in the following pages.
- Stay active and get on with your life.

Some people have more persistent pain – but the same principles apply.

Control of pain

There are many treatments that can help - even if there is no miracle cure. They may not remove the pain completely, but they should control it enough to let you get moving and active. They do not solve the problem. Your body does that – with your help.

Pain killers

You should not hesitate to use painkillers if you need them. You can safely mask the pain to get active: your body will not let you do any harm. Paracetamol is the simplest and safest pain killer, or you can use anti-inflammatory tablets like Ibuprofen.

It may surprise you, but these simple over-the-counter painkillers are often the most effective for neck pain. The problem is that many people don't use them properly. You should take the full recommended dose and take them regularly every 4-6 hours - do not wait till your pain is out of control. You should usually take the painkillers for a few days, but you may need to take them for a week or two. Few people require anything stronger. Do not take Ibuprofen or Aspirin if you are pregnant, if you have asthma, or if you have indigestion or have had an ulcer.

Collars

Collars used to be given to support the neck, but the problem was that it stopped your neck moving. New research shows they do not help long-term. You'll get better faster if you do without a collar.

Heat & cold

Heat or cold can be used for short-term relief of pain and to relax muscle tension. In the first 48 hours you can try a cold pack on the sore area for 5-10 minutes at a time - a bag of frozen peas wrapped in a damp towel. Other people prefer heat - a hot water bottle, a bath, or a shower.

Massage

Massage is one of the oldest treatments for neck pain. Many people find simple rubbing eases the pain and relaxes muscle spasm.

Manipulation

Most doctors now agree that manipulation can help neck pain. It is safe if done by a qualified professional: osteopaths, chiropractors, some physiotherapists and a few doctors with special training. It is probably most effective in the early stages, and can help you get active. You should begin to feel the benefit within a few sessions. It's not a good idea to have treatment for weeks and months on end.

Other treatments

Many other treatments such as electro-therapy machines, acupuncture, or alternative medicine are used for neck pain and some people feel they help. But be realistic. Despite the claims, these treatments rarely provide a quick fix. Once again, you should feel any benefit quite quickly and there is no value in treatment for months on end. What really matters is whether they help you get active.

EXERCISES

Exercise is good for neck pain and it's a way to treat yourself. Simple neck exercises are safe and effective. They reduce the pain and help you get on with your life. They get your neck moving again by stretching tight muscles and joints, and prevent the working parts from stiffening up. Don't worry if they make you a bit sore to start with. It's the improvement in function that's important, because once you get full movement and are back to full activity the pain should ease off.

There is no single exercise that is right for everyone. So don't be afraid to experiment to find what works best for you and your neck. You should always do neck exercises slowly and regularly.
Move to the point of pain, then gradually try to go a little bit further each time.

To give you an idea of the sort of exercises you can do yourself, here are some suggestions to get you started. Obviously you need to exercise your neck, but it also helps to work your shoulders. You can exercise sitting or standing, or if that's too painful you could try some of them lying on your back. Or you might find it easier to start when your muscles are warm, perhaps after or even during a hot shower.

Do the exercises slowly, taking about 5 seconds to move in each direction. Aim to do each movement at least 2-3 times, several times a day.

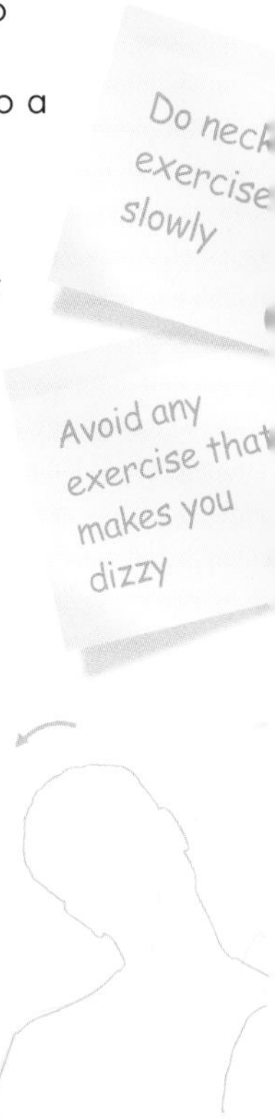

If your pain seems worse, do them slower and through a smaller range, rather than stop altogether. Then as the pain eases you can build up again. You should avoid rolling your head around. The exercises should not cause other symptoms - if a particular exercise causes dizziness, or tingling/numbness/weakness in your hands you should try a different one.

Neck stretching

You need to move your head slowly in each direction – forwards and backwards, leaning over to both sides and turning your head right and left. Move your head in one direction then in the opposite direction as far as you feel you can.

Shoulder stretching

Moving your arms stretches your shoulder muscles –

- Shrug your shoulders while breathing in and then relax them whilst breathing out. Try rolling them at the same time.
- Circle your arms, one at a time, backwards and forwards – like swimming crawl and backstroke. Bend the elbows if that's easier.

Neck strengthening

You should also do some strengthening exercises. These will help you get safely back to normal activity, and help control posture.

The idea is to make your neck muscles work without actually moving your head. Put your hand on the side of your head and apply increasing pressure. As you resist, you will feel your muscles contracting. Maintain the force for 10 seconds and then gradually release. Repeat to the other side. Similarly, push forwards against both hands on your forehead, and then backwards against your clasped hands behind your head.

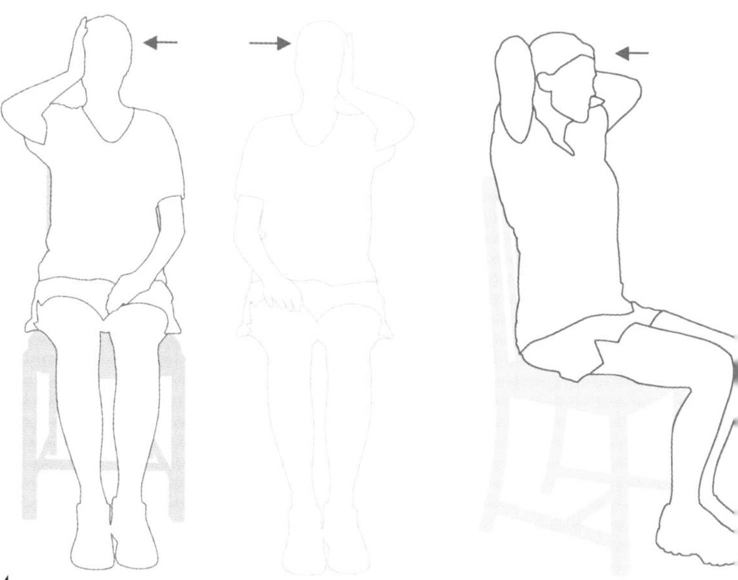

Posture

Some people find it helps to control their neck posture. A common problem is letting your head poke forwards. Instead you should 'walk tall', trying to keep your chin in. Let your shoulders relax, rather than hunched up. This should help you feel better, and you'll look more normal!

If you need extra help you could see a physiotherapist, who is an expert on exercise and rehabilitation. But physiotherapists can't do the exercises for you. They may show you how and help you to get started, but you have to put in the effort and do the work yourself. So the sooner you are doing the exercises yourself the better. And once again there's no value in going for treatment for months on end.

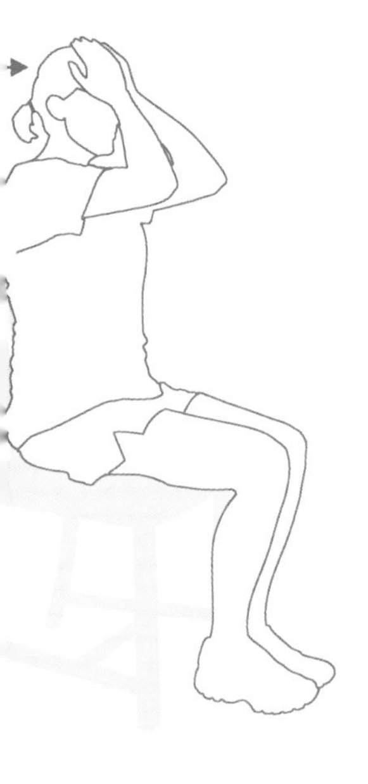

ANXIETY, STRESS, AND MUSCLE TENSION

Anyone who has neck problems will tell you that pain causes stress. Anxiety and stress can also make pain feel worse. Tension can cause muscle spasm and the muscles themselves can become painful - we have all had a tension headache. This can produce a vicious circle.

It's natural to get anxious about neck pain, especially if it doesn't get better as fast as you expect. You may get conflicting advice - from your family and friends or even from doctors and therapists - which may make you uncertain what best to do. Trust the advice in this booklet - it comes from the latest research.

Stress creates tension, and can aggravate or prolong pain. If stress is a problem you need to recognise it at an early stage and try to do something about it. You cannot always avoid stress, but you can learn to reduce its effects by controlled breathing, muscle relaxation, and mental calming techniques.

Relaxation

Lie comfortably on your back with eyes closed knees bent up over a pillow.
The idea is to contract each set of muscles and then let them go – starting with your toes, working up to your neck. Simply spending a few minutes doing this throughout the body will ease muscle tension and reduce stress.

also:

Lying in the same position, simply breathe in slowly through the nose and feel your abdomen rise – breath out through your mouth and feel your abdomen gently fall. Try this for a few minutes – some people fall asleep!

One of the best ways of reducing stress and tension is exercise. Though relaxation and exercises are different, many people find that both can help control neck pain. You need to find what works best for you. Or you might use them at different times.

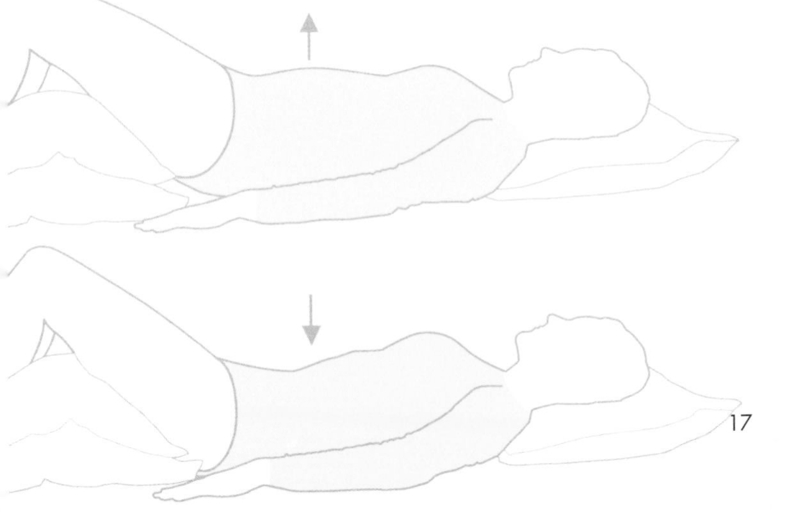

THE RISK OF CHRONIC PAIN

There has been a lot of recent research to find who is at risk of long-term pain and disability. What may surprise you is that most of the warning signs are about what people feel and do, rather than medical findings.

Signs of people at risk of long-term pain:

- Believing that you have a serious injury or damage. Being unable to accept reassurance.
- Believing that hurt means harm and that you will become disabled.
- Avoiding movement or activity due to fear of doing damage.
- Continued rest and inactivity instead of getting on with your life.
- Waiting for someone to fix it rather than believing that you can help yourself recover.
- Becoming withdrawn and depressed.

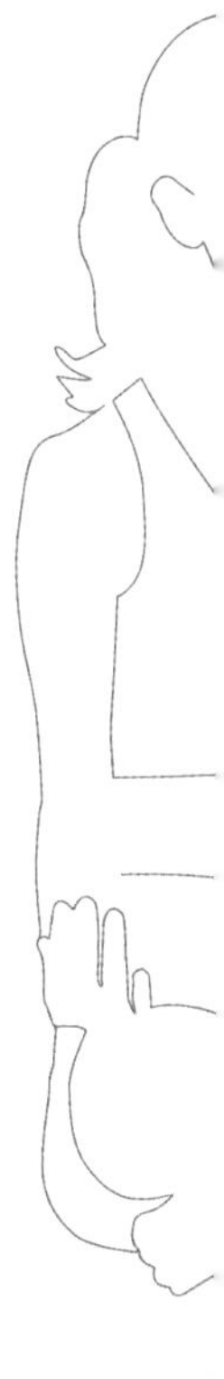

This all develops gradually and you may not even notice. That's why it is so important to get going as soon as possible *before* you develop chronic pain. If you - or your family and friends - spot some of these early warning signs, you need to do something about it. Now, before it is too late. Use the advice in this booklet to work out what you can do to change direction and get on with your life. If you need extra help to get going, you should ask your doctor or therapist.

You may meet a practical problem here. Doctors and therapists deal best with clear-cut diseases and injuries for which they have a cure. We are often not so good at dealing with more ordinary symptoms like neck pain. For example, it's no good staying off work and doing nothing for weeks on end to attend therapy. That simply delays your recovery! Which is why it really does depend on what you do yourself. You should make it clear to your doctor or therapist that you realise all this, and what you want is help to get on with your life.

If you are still off work after about a month, you are at risk of developing long-term problems. There is then a 10% risk you will still be off work in a year's time. You could even lose your job. Long before you get to that stage you really need to face up to the problem and take urgent action.

HOW TO STAY ACTIVE

Doctors, physiotherapists, chiropractors and osteopaths all agree: the sooner you start getting mobile and active again the better. It's worth working through any initial discomfort – because you'll get back to normal that much quicker. Of course, you may need to take it a little easier or do some things more carefully at first. But don't stop altogether.

Fortunately, you don't need a fully mobile neck to do most of the things you want to do. You can do most daily activities if you think about them first or change the way you do them. Work out a plan. What are the problems and how can you get round them? Can you do things a different way?

The idea is to strike a balance between being as active as you can and not putting too much strain on your neck – just use common sense!

- Keep moving.
- Do not stay in one position for too long.
- Move about before you stiffen up.
- Don't stop doing things - just change the way you do them.

Sitting	Choose a chair and position that is comfortable for you - experiment. Get up regularly – take advantage of TV adverts!
Driving	Adjust your seat so that you can hold the steering wheel comfortably. Stop regularly for a few minutes break - get out of the car and walk about. If reversing is a problem, just turn your head slower or use the mirrors.
Desk work	Adjust the height of your chair to suit your desk. Adjust your keyboard and screen so that your neck and shoulders are comfortable. Keep the mouse close. Don't look down for too long. Avoid jamming the phone between shoulder and ear! Get up and stretch regularly.
Arm use at work	Take regular short breaks from forceful or repetitive work. Adjust your position - work with your arms low. Get close to things - avoid awkward reaching.
Carrying and shopping	Think if you need to carry at all. Carry things hugged to your body or split the load between both hands. Use wheels!
Daily activities and hobbies	Do each activity for a short period. Keep changing activities. Use your arms at or below shoulder level. Don't tilt your head back for too long.
Sports	Continuing with your normal sports is fine if it's non-impact or non-contact. Just reduce the intensity for a while, if you need to. Swimming - try a different stroke – backstroke, sidestroke.
Sleeping	Your head and neck should be comfortable. Find what pillow is best for you – higher or lower, softer or firmer – maybe a different shape helps. Experiment! Try taking painkillers an hour before you go to bed.

GETTING ON WITH YOUR LIFE

It is important to maintain the momentum of your life - and that includes staying at work if you possibly can. Doing things will distract you from the pain, and your neck will usually not get any worse at work than it will at home. If some of your job tasks put a lot of strain on your neck and shoulders, you may need some help from your work mates. Simple changes may make your job easier. The main thing is to have a brief break every 20 minutes or so.

If you are seeing a doctor or therapist, tell them about your work. Talk to your supervisor or boss if you need to. Tell them about any parts of your job that may be difficult to begin with, but stress that you want to be at work. Offer your own suggestions about how to overcome these problems - you might even show them this booklet.

If you do have to stay off work, it helps to get back as soon as possible – usually within days or a couple of weeks - and even if you still have some pain. The longer you are inactive and off work the more likely you are to develop long-term pain and disability.

If you are not at work within about a month you should be planning with your doctor, therapist and employer how and when you can get back. Your occupational health department or health and safety rep may be able to assist. Temporary modification to your job or pattern of work may help you get back sooner.

WHAT DOCTORS CAN AND CAN'T DO

Although we have stressed that you can deal with most neck pain yourself, there may be times you are uncertain and feel the need to check. That's reasonable. But remember there is no quick fix for neck pain. So you should be realistic about what you expect from your doctor or therapist.They can:

- Make sure you don't have any serious disease and reassure you.
- Suggest various treatments to help control your pain.
- Advise you on how you can best deal with the pain and get on with your life.

Try to accept the reassurance and don't let needless worry delay your recovery. You have to share responsibility for your own progress. Some doctors and therapists may be hesitant about handing over and letting you take control. You may have to tell them straight out this really is what you want.

Doctors and therapists can help to ease the pain but only you can get your neck going!

Warning signs

If you have severe pain that is getting worse instead of better, or if you are unwell with neck pain, you should see your doctor.

Here are a few symptoms, which are all very rare, but if you do have neck pain and develop any of these you should see a doctor straight away.

- Lumps or swelling in your neck
- Difficulty swallowing
- Difficulty breathing
- Dizziness or fainting
- Difficulty lifting your arm, dropping things, or clumsiness in your fingers
- Falling, tripping or dragging your feet

Don't let that list worry you too much.

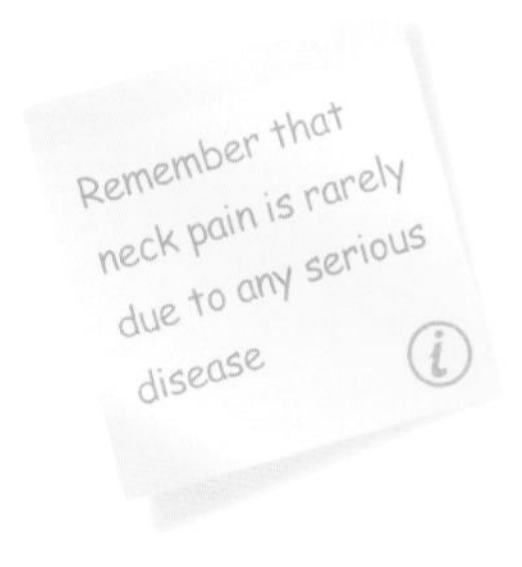

IT'S YOUR NECK

We've shown you that neck pain is rarely due to anything serious and it should not disable you unless you let it. You've got the facts and the most up-to-date advice about how to deal with neck pain. The important thing now is for you to get on with your life. How your neck affects you depends on how you react to the pain and what you do about it yourself.

There is no instant answer. You will have your ups and downs - that's normal. But look at it this way:

There are two types of sufferer

☹ One who *avoids* activity
☺ and one who *copes*

☹ The avoider gets frightened by the pain and worries about the future.

- The avoider is afraid that hurting always means further damage - it doesn't.
- The avoider rests a lot, and just waits for the pain to get better.

☺ The coper knows that the pain will get better and does not fear the future.

- The coper carries on as normally as possible.
- The coper deals with the pain by being positive, staying active and getting on with life.

Who suffers most?

☹ Avoiders suffer the most. They have pain for longer, they have more time off work and they can become disabled.

☺ Copers get better faster, enjoy life more and have less trouble in the long run.

So how do I become a Coper and prevent unnecessary suffering?

Follow these guidelines - you really can help yourself.

☺ Live life as normally as possible. This is much better than giving in to the pain.

- Keep up daily activities - they will not cause damage. Just avoid really heavy things.
- Try to stay fit - even after your neck feels better.
- Start gradually and do a little more each day so you can see the progress you are making.
- Either stay at work or go back to work as soon as possible. If necessary, ask if you can get lighter or modified duties for a week or two.
- Be patient. It's normal to get aches or twinges for a time.

☹ Don't rely on painkillers alone. Stay positive and take control of the pain yourself.

- Don't stay at home or give up doing things you enjoy.

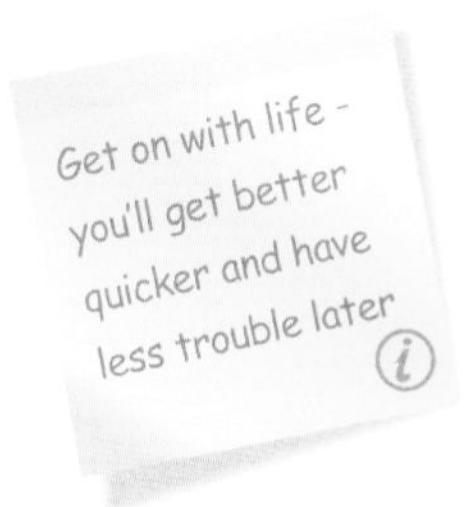